Sweet Serenade :

Glucose World Exploration"

By

Vernon B. Hopkins

Disclaimer

Copyright © by Vernon B. Hopkins 2023. All rights reserved.
Before this document is duplicated or reproduced in any manner, the publisher's consent must be gained. Therefore, the contents within can neither be stored electronically, transferred, nor kept in a database. Neither in Part nor full can the document be copied, scanned, faxed, or retained without approval from the publisher or creator.

Table of contents

Description
Introduction:
Chapter 1: The Essence of Sweetness
Chapter 2: A Trip to Nature's Pantry
Chapter 3: From Farm to Fork
Chapter 4: Fueling Our Cells
Chapter 5: Sweet Science
Chapter 6: The Dark Side of Sweetness
Chapter 7: Beyond the Palate
Chapter 8: The Sweet Symphony of Flavors
Chapter 8: The Sweet Symphony of Flavors
Chapter 9: The Cultural Connection
Conclusion.

Description

"Sweet Serenade: Exploring the World of Glucose" transports readers to the fascinating and beautiful world of glucose. This engrossing book goes deeply into the core of sweetness, revealing the molecular structure and characteristics of glucose as well as its interesting position as an important energy source inside the human body.

This book explores the natural sources of glucose, such as fruits, vegetables, and honey, from nature's abundant pantry to our plates. It delves into the delicate process of photosynthesis, offering insight into how plants create glucose and how it appears in different civilizations via their culinary traditions.

The voyage of glucose from farm to fork continues as the book dives into the various harvesting and processing procedures used to get glucose-rich crops to our meals. Readers acquire a better grasp of the influence of food processing on glucose levels, allowing them to make more educated dietary decisions.

The book, Unlocking the Secrets of Glucose Metabolism, sheds insight on its critical function in feeding our cells. It unravels the relevance of glucose in brain function and cognitive functions by navigating the complicated interaction between glucose and insulin. It digs into the chemistry of glucose in food preparation, cooking, and preservation with scientific accuracy, improving readers' comprehension of its transformational function in numerous culinary creations.

"Sweet Serenade" does not, however, shy away from confronting the evil side of sweetness. It investigates the complex relationships between obesity, diabetes, and other metabolic illnesses to provide light on the health consequences of excessive glucose intake. Readers get vital insights and solutions for balancing their glucose consumption and promoting general well-being.

But the influence of glucose extends beyond the taste, and this book bravely delves into the non-edible uses of glucose in a variety of sectors. It demonstrates its critical role in medications, cosmetics, and even biofuels, highlighting the vast potential and intriguing discoveries on the horizon.

"Sweet Serenade" highlights flavor creativity by delving into the harmonic harmony formed when glucose meets culinary expertise. Readers are encouraged to try and improve their culinary talents with tasty recipes, insightful hints, and fascinating tales.

Furthermore, this cultural journey links readers to the rich fabric of human history and its connection to glucose. The book explores how glucose has affected and altered cultural identities and practices across the globe, from ancient civilizations to current society.

"Sweet Serenade: Exploring the World of Glucose" is an engrossing inquiry that enlightens, inspires, and deepens the reader's knowledge of glucose—a little molecule with an enormous impact on our lives.

Introduction:

Welcome to "Sweet Serenade: Exploring the World of Glucose," a riveting trip into the enthralling world of one of nature's most enthralling compounds. Glucose, an innocuous sugar, hides a symphony of mysteries waiting to be discovered. This book takes you on an examination of glucose that will leave you enthralled and informed, from its chemical structure to its tremendous influence on our bodies and culinary creations.

In the pages that follow, we'll go through the essence of sweetness, delving deep into the chemistry and features of glucose. We shall discover the complicated network of connections between glucose and our health, societies, and even our planet as a whole.

Nature's pantry is brimming with glucose-rich foods, and we'll explore their many expressions across countries and civilizations. From the delectable fruits that tempt our taste buds to the golden nectar of honey, we will investigate nature's abundance and the distinct flavors that result from the presence of glucose.

But our investigation does not end with harvest. We'll trace glucose's trip from the fields to our plates, delving into the intriguing processes and strategies that make it possible. We will investigate the transformational stages that change the availability and effect of glucose in our diets, from agricultural practices to food processing.

We shall discover the fundamental significance that glucose plays in feeding our cells and energizing our bodies as we dive further into its metabolic pathways. We shall unravel the secrets of glucose's fundamental contributions to human well-being, from the complicated dance between glucose and insulin to the critical significance of glucose in brain function.

However, like with any compelling story, our investigation must also explore the shadows that accompany sweetness. We will discuss the health consequences of high glucose intake, focusing on the relationships between glucose and obesity, diabetes, and other metabolic problems. We will empower ourselves to make educated decisions and cultivate a harmonious relationship with this potent chemical by increasing our understanding and awareness.

However, the influence of glucose goes well beyond the limitations of our bodies. We will investigate its non-edible uses, learning about its multifaceted function in sectors like medicines, cosmetics, and even biofuels. Witness the incredible possibilities and fascinating breakthroughs that occur when glucose meets science and technology.

Prepare to be tempted as we investigate the craftsmanship of flavors. From the chemistry of glucose in food preparation to the sumptuous realm of pastries and sweets, we will see how this modest sugar can alter. We welcome you to embrace your inner culinary maestro and take your creations to new heights with a variety of recipes, ideas, and tactics.

We will construct a tapestry of cultural links throughout our journey, charting the impact of glucose on human history and rituals. Join us as we celebrate the unique culinary legacy that results from the presence of glucose, as well as the cultural importance that it carries for communities throughout the world.

So take a seat and be ready for an incredible voyage into the world of glucose. "Sweet Serenade" is ready to enchant your senses, broaden your understanding, and leave you with a new appreciation for the lovely symphony that glucose orchestrates in our life.

Chapter 1: The Essence of Sweetness

Understanding the chemical structure and properties of glucose

Glucose is a simple sugar that belongs to the carbohydrate family and is classed as a monosaccharide. It is an important chemical in biology and a major source of energy for living creatures. Let's look at the molecular structure and characteristics of glucose to have a better grasp of its intriguing qualities.

The chemical formula for glucose, often known as dextrose, is C6H12O6. There are six carbon atoms (C6), twelve hydrogen atoms (H12), and six oxygen atoms (O6) in it. Glucose molecules have a ring structure, particularly a hexagonal ring, making it a six-carbon sugar.

Glucose may be found in two structural forms: -glucose and -glucose isomers. The orientation of the hydroxyl group (OH) linked to the first carbon atom (C1) of the glucose molecule differs between these isomers. The hydroxyl group in -glucose points downwards, while it points upwards in -glucose. This small structural diversity gives birth to unique characteristics and biological activities.

1. Solubility: Due to its hydrophilic nature, glucose is extremely soluble in water. It generates large hydrogen bonds with water molecules, which allows it to dissolve quickly and produce a stable aqueous solution.

2. Sweetness: Glucose has a sweet taste, which contributes to the overall sense of sweetness in a variety of meals and drinks. It has a mild sweetness when compared to other sugars, but it is an important component of the overall flavor profile.

3. Stability: Glucose is relatively stable, particularly when dry. It may, however, undergo reactions when exposed to heat, acids, or enzymes. The Maillard reaction, which happens when glucose combines with amino acids and results in browning and the creation of attractive flavors and fragrances in cooked meals, is one prominent process.

4. Reducing Sugar: Because of its propensity to contribute electrons in chemical processes, glucose is classed as reducing sugar. It may decrease other chemicals due to the presence of an aldehyde group (-CHO) in its structure. This feature is important in many biological processes including food chemistry.

5. Energy Source: Glucose is an essential energy source for all living species, including humans. During cellular respiration, glucose undergoes metabolic reactions that result in the production of adenosine triphosphate (ATP), the cell's energy currency. Glucose molecules are broken down in a sequence of processes, generating energy that supports cellular activity.

6. Biochemical Role: Glucose plays an important role in various metabolic processes, including glycolysis, gluconeogenesis, and glycogenesis. It acts as a precursor for the production of other biomolecules like glycogen, nucleotides, and fatty acids, and hence contributes to a variety of physiological processes.

Understanding glucose's chemical structure and characteristics lays the groundwork for understanding its critical function in biology, nutrition, and food science. Its distinct structure and properties make it an interesting molecule to investigate and admire.

The role of glucose in the human body and its significance as an energy source

Glucose is a crucial energy source in the human body. It is the major fuel for many physiological activities and is especially important for giving energy to the brain, muscles, and other tissues. Let's look at the importance of glucose as an energy source and its role in sustaining general biological processes.

1. Energy Production: Glucose is the preferred energy source for most cells in the body. In the cytoplasm of cells, glucose is broken down by a sequence of metabolic events known as glycolysis. This mechanism transforms glucose into pyruvate, producing a little quantity of ATP (adenosine triphosphate), the cellular energy currency. Pyruvate may then be further metabolized by aerobic respiration in the presence of oxygen or transformed into lactate under anaerobic circumstances.

2. Brain Function: Glucose is critical to brain function. Unlike other organs, the brain depends largely on glucose as its principal energy source. Despite accounting for just around 2% of the body's weight, it contributes to roughly 20% of total glucose utilization. Neurons in the brain

need a steady supply of glucose to sustain electrical activity and conduct important cognitive processes.

3. Muscle Contraction: Glucose is necessary for muscle contraction. Muscles need significant amounts of energy to contract and do work during physical effort or exercise. Glucose stored in the muscles as glycogen may be swiftly degraded into glucose molecules, providing the required fuel for muscular activity. Glucose from the circulation may also be taken up by muscle cells to satisfy their energy needs.

4. Blood Sugar Level Maintenance: Glucose regulation in the body is strictly managed to maintain stable blood sugar levels. The pancreatic hormone insulin regulates glucose metabolism. When blood glucose levels are high, such as after a meal, insulin promotes glucose absorption into cells, especially muscle and adipose tissue, where it may be utilized for energy or stored as glycogen. During fasting or in between meals, the liver may release stored glucose (through glycogenolysis) into the circulation to maintain glucose levels and offer a consistent supply of energy to numerous organs.

5. Energy for Cellular Processes: Glucose is a crucial building ingredient for many biomolecules. It may be transformed into intermediates used in the production of amino acids, nucleotides, and fatty acids. These biomolecules are essential for cellular development, repair, and maintenance, as well as the appropriate function of tissues and organs.

Overall, glucose's importance as an energy source in the human body cannot be emphasized. It fuels key activities, promotes brain function, allows muscular contraction, regulates blood sugar levels, and acts as a precursor for the creation of essential proteins. Without an appropriate supply of glucose, the body's metabolic activities and general well-being would be significantly hampered.

Exploring the taste and perception of sweetness

Exploring the taste and perception of sweetness gives a wonderful insight into the complicated realm of flavor. Let us dig into the fascinating world of sweetness, investigating its sensory perception and the aspects that contribute to our enjoyment of this delectable flavor.

1. Taste Receptors: Our capacity to feel sweetness is based on specialized taste receptors found in our taste buds. These sweet taste receptors are proteins that are found on the surface of taste cells. When molecules with sweet qualities interact with these receptors, they set off a chain reaction of biochemical signals that cause the experience of sweetness.

2. Sweetness Threshold: Everyone has a different sensitivity to sweetness, with different thresholds for perceiving sweet taste. Some individuals have heightened sensitivity to sweetness and may detect it even at low doses, whilst others may need larger quantities to have the same sensation. Individuals' perceptions of sweetness may be influenced by genetic variables and earlier exposure to sweet stimuli.

3. sense of Sweet Taste: The sense of sweetness is not only reliant on the presence of sugars such as glucose or fructose. A variety of chemicals, including artificial sweeteners like aspartame and natural compounds like stevia, may elicit a sweet taste experience. Each sweet chemical interacts with distinct sweet taste receptors, stimulating sweetness perception in diverse ways.

4. Synergy and Taste Modulation: Other taste experiences may increase or modify sweetness. For example, the presence of sourness or bitterness at the same time might inhibit or hide the impression of sweetness. The sweetness combined with particular flavors, such as fruity or creamy overtones, on the other hand, may provide a more satisfying and well-rounded taste experience.

5. Cultural and Individual Differences: Cultural and individual differences may also alter the sense of sweetness. Different cultures have different sweetening preferences in their traditional meals and drinks. Furthermore, an individual's perception and taste for sweetness may be shaped by personal experiences, dietary habits, and even age.

6. Emotional and Hedonic aspects: Sweetness is more than just a sensory experience; it also has emotional and hedonic aspects. It is often connected with happiness and joy. Endorphins and dopamine are released in reaction to sweet tastes, which adds to pleasure experiences and encourages the desire for sweet meals.

7. situation and Expectations: The situation in which sweetness is encountered may have a significant influence on its perception. A meal or beverage's setting, presentation, and even labeling may all impact our expectations and how we experience its sweetness. Aesthetic appeal, temperature, and the presence of other flavors may all influence how we perceive flavor.

Exploring the taste and perception of sweetness shows a complex interaction between our sensory systems, biology, culture, and personal preferences. Understanding these variables not only broadens our appreciation for sweetness in our lives but also provides insights into the fascinating realm of flavor perception and its tremendous impact on our culinary choices and pleasure.

Chapter 2: A Trip to Nature's Pantry

Unveiling the natural sources of glucose: fruits, vegetables, and honey

Uncovering the natural sources of glucose leads us through the bright world of fruits and vegetables, as well as the golden nectar of honey. These many sources provide a wide range of flavors, nutrients, and the sweet taste of glucose. Let us investigate these natural riches and learn about the many ways they contribute to our culinary experiences and general well-being.

1. Fruits: Nature's culinary gems, and fruits provide a delectable array of flavors and textures, each with its unique mix of nutrients and glucose content. Fruits, from luscious berries to juicy citrus fruits and tropical treats, not only give natural sweetness but also a variety of vitamins, minerals, and fiber. Fruits containing considerable levels of glucose, such as bananas, apples, grapes, and mangoes, are a delightful and energizing snack choice.

2. veggies: While veggies aren't often linked with sweetness, some types do add to our glucose consumption. Because of their high glucose content, root vegetables such as sweet potatoes and carrots have a naturally sweet flavor. These nutritional jewels provide a combination of complex carbs, vitamins, and minerals, making them useful complements to savory recipes and adding a delicate sweetness to culinary masterpieces.

3. Honey: Honey, revered for its golden color and enticing flavor, is a magnificent natural sweetener produced by bees from floral nectar. It is mostly constituted of glucose and fructose, giving it a distinct and complex flavor character. Honey has long been prized for its purported therapeutic powers as well as its function in improving the flavor of meals and drinks. Because of its flexibility in both sweet and savory uses, it is a prized ingredient in culinary traditions all across the globe.

These natural sources of glucose not only sweeten our palates but also provide a plethora of health advantages. Fruits and vegetables include vital vitamins, minerals, antioxidants, and dietary fiber, which promote general health and support a variety of biological activities. Their natural glucose content provides a source of long-lasting energy, making them a nutritious option for active people.

It is important to note that consuming these natural sources of glucose should be part of a well-balanced and diverse diet. While glucose is an important energy source, an excess of intense sweets, even natural sources, may lead to calorie overconsumption. The key to receiving the advantages of these natural sources while maintaining a healthy lifestyle is moderation and attentive eating.

We celebrate the balance between flavor and nutrition by embracing the natural sweetness of fruits, vegetables, and honey. These natural gifts not only tempt our taste senses but also fuel our bodies, reminding us of the vast and plentiful offers of the natural world. So, as you go on a tour through the natural sources of glucose, savor the lusciousness of fruits, the delicate sweetness of vegetables, and the golden essence of honey.

The process of photosynthesis and glucose production in plants

Photosynthesis is an amazing biological process that happens in plants, algae, and certain microorganisms. It is in charge of turning solar energy into chemical energy in the form of glucose. Let's look at the intriguing process of photosynthesis and how it leads to the generation of glucose in plants.

1. Sunlight Absorption: Photosynthesis starts with the absorption of sunlight by specialized pigments called chlorophyll, which are found in plant cells' chloroplasts. Chlorophyll absorbs light in the red and blue parts of the electromagnetic spectrum while reflecting green light, resulting in plants' distinctive green color.

2. Light Energy Conversion: The absorbed solar energy is used to fuel a series of complicated chemical processes. Light energy is turned into chemical energy in the form of adenosine triphosphate (ATP) and another energy carrier molecule known as nicotinamide adenine dinucleotide phosphate (NADPH) throughout this process. These energy-dense molecules serve as fuel for future processes.

3. Carbon Dioxide Uptake: Plants absorb carbon dioxide (CO_2) from the atmosphere through minute holes called stomata, which are mostly found on the leaves. Carbon dioxide molecules infiltrate into plant cells, where they may be processed further.

4. The Calvin Cycle: The collected energy in the form of ATP and NADPH is used in the chloroplasts in a series of enzyme processes known as the Calvin cycle. The Calvin cycle is in charge of fixing carbon dioxide and eventually creating glucose.

5. Carbon Fixation: Using an enzyme called RuBisCO, carbon dioxide molecules join with a five-carbon complex called ribulose-1,5-bisphosphate (RuBP) in the first phase of the Calvin cycle. This reaction produces two three-carbon molecules known as 3-phosphoglycerate (3-PGA).

6. Reduction and Conversion: The ATP and NADPH produced in step 2 by the light-dependent processes are used to reduce and convert the 3-PGA molecules. The energy carriers supply electrons and energy via a series of enzymatic processes, eventually transforming the 3-PGA molecules into a three-carbon sugar known as glyceraldehyde-3-phosphate (G3P).

7. Glucose Formation: Some of the G3P molecules created in the Calvin cycle are utilized o renew RuBP, which ensures the cycle's continuance. However, some G3P molecules are devoted to the production of glucose and other carbohydrates. These molecules may unite and undergo further enzymatic activities, yielding glucose, the major carbohydrate product of photosynthesis.

8. Energy Storage: Glucose, which is created during photosynthesis, is an important energy storage molecule in plants. It may be transformed into different forms for long-term energy storage, such as starch or cellulose, or consumed for immediate energy demands through cellular respiration.

Photosynthesis not only creates glucose but also has a significant influence on our world. It is in charge of producing oxygen, altering the Earth's atmosphere, and maintaining a variety of habitats. In addition, photosynthesis is important in the carbon cycle because it helps to control global temperature patterns by eliminating carbon dioxide from the atmosphere.

Understanding photosynthesis and glucose production in plants reveals the complex link between plants, sunlight, and energy conversion. It demonstrates plants' incredible capacity to capture the power of sunlight and turn it into glucose, a critical energy-rich chemical on which many species, including humans, depend for nourishment and life.

Exploring the diversity of glucose-rich foods across cultures

The diversity of glucose-rich meals seen in different countries mirrors the amazing variety of culinary traditions and ingredients found across the world. Glucose, a fundamental source of energy, may be found in a wide range of foods that reflect the diverse tastes, techniques, and cultural histories of many regions. Let us go on a journey to uncover the rich tapestry of glucose-rich meals found in different cuisines throughout the globe.

1. Rice-based Delights (Asia): Rice is a staple carbohydrate and a rich source of glucose in many Asian countries. Rice is the foundation of many regional cuisines, from Thai fragrant jasmine rice to Southeast Asian sticky rice delights. Glutinous rice cakes, rice puddings, and rice-based confections such as mochi show how glucose-rich rice may be transformed into delicious sweets in unique ways.

2. European Sweet Pastries and Sweets: A delightful range of glucose-rich pastries and sweets may be found in European cuisines. From flaky croissants and pain au chocolat in France to creamy pastries like cannoli in Italy and sumptuous cakes like Black Forest cake in Germany, these beautiful delicacies often include ingredients like wheat, butter, sugar, and fruits, all of which contribute to their glucose content.

3. Middle Eastern Sweets: Middle Eastern cuisine has a wide selection of tasty glucose-rich sweets. The region is well-known for using ingredients including dates, honey, nuts, and aromatic spices to create delightful desserts such as baklava, kunafa, halva, and Turkish delight. These sweets have a nice texture and taste combination, frequently combining sweetness with nuttiness or floral undertones.

4. Tropical Fruits (Latin America and the Caribbean): The tropical regions of Latin America and the Caribbean are home to a wealth of glucose-rich fruits that are delicious. Mangoes, pineapples, bananas, papayas, and passion fruits are just a few of the tasty fruits eaten in these civilizations. When eaten fresh, in fruit salads, or desserts like flan or tropical fruit sorbets, these fruits provide both sweetness and refreshing qualities.

5. Indigenous Staples (Africa): Traditional staples like yams, plantains, and millet play a critical role in supplying glucose-rich meals throughout Africa's many geographies. These ingredients may be found in a variety of meals, including stews, porridges, and fritters. Fufu, a dough-like delicacy made from starchy root vegetables, is a common accompaniment to savory dishes in West Africa, for example.

6. Traditional Sweeteners (Global): Aside from the natural glucose found in many foods, countries throughout the world have developed their traditional sweeteners. All-natural plant-based sweeteners include maple syrup in North America, jaggery in South Asia, agave nectar in Mexico, and palm sugar in Southeast Asia. These sweeteners, which are rich in glucose and other sugars, are used to flavor meals and beverages in regional cuisines.

Exploring the ethnic diversity of glucose-rich meals reveals the incredible depth and ingenuity of culinary traditions all around the world. These cuisines provide sustenance while also commemorating cultural heritage, expressing creativity, and bringing people together. Whether they are rice-based delicacies, sweet pastries, tropical fruits, or indigenous staples, glucose-rich meals ambo symbolize specific tastes and experiences that define each culture's cuisine.

Chapter 3: From Farm to Fork

The journey of glucose from agricultural fields to our plates

From agricultural fields to our plates, glucose travels via a complicated and interrelated process that includes production, harvest, processing, distribution, and culinary preparation. Let's follow glucose on its wonderful trip to our plates, where it nourishes us with energy and contributes to the flavors and textures of our meals.

1. Agricultural Cultivation: The voyage starts in agricultural areas, where farmers grow glucose-rich crops. Glucose may be obtained from a variety of plants, including cereal crops such as rice, wheat, and maize, as well as fruits, vegetables, and tubers. Farmers tend to these crops carefully, ensuring ideal growth conditions via irrigation, fertilization, insect control, and other agricultural practices.

2. Harvesting: When crops reach maturity, farmers or farm laborers harvest them. Harvesting techniques vary depending on the crop but might involve human picking, machine harvesting, or a mix of the two. Because glucose levels fluctuate at various phases of plant development, harvest time is critical to ensuring optimum sugar content and crop quality.

3. Extraction and processing: Once harvested, the crops are processed to extract or refine glucose. In the case of cereal crops such as rice or wheat, milling or grinding techniques may be used to separate the outer husk from the starchy endosperm, which contains glucose-rich carbohydrates. Fruits and vegetables are often cleaned, sorted, and processed o extract the naturally occurring sugars in their pulp or juice.

4. Sugar Production: Some crops, such as sugarcane or sugar beets, require specialized processing to generate refined sugar. Sugarcane is crushed to obtain its juice, which is then concentrated by filtration, clarifying, and evaporation procedures. Sugar beets are similarly cut, and their juice is collected and processed to produce refined sugar crystals.

5. Distribution and Supply Chain: Once processed, glucose-rich crops, extracts, or refined sugar are carried via the supply chain at different stages. Distribution to processing facilities, wholesalers, distributors, and retailers is required to make the goods accessible to consumers. Quality control methods, packaging, and labeling are undertaken along the route to assure the safety and integrity of glucose-containing goods.

6. Culinary Preparation: Finally, glucose-rich substances or products are used in culinary preparations in our homes or at professional food outlets. Glucose may be found in a variety of recipes and cuisines, whether in the form of fresh fruits and vegetables, grains, sugars, or sweeteners. It is used in baking, confectionery, sweet sauces, drinks, and a variety of other culinary creations to add sweetness, texture, and vitality to our meals.

The journey of glucose from agricultural fields to our plates emphasizes the food system's interdependence, which includes farmers, processors, distributors, and consumers. It focuses on the complicated procedures and partnerships required to deliver this vital energy source to our meals. We savor the conclusion of hard effort, skill, and nature's abundance with each meal, enjoying the journey that feeds and supports us.

Harvesting and processing techniques of glucose-rich crops

Harvesting and processing methods for glucose-rich crops differ depending on the product and its intended application. Let's look at some of the most prevalent procedures for harvesting and preparing various kinds of glucose-rich crops.

1. Cereals (Rice, Wheat, and Corn):
- Gathering: Cereal crops such as rice, wheat, and maize are normally harvested at maturity. Harvesting at the right time is critical to ensuring adequate sugar content. For efficiency, mechanical harvesting techniques like combine harvesters are often utilized. Cut, collected, and separated from the plant are the crops.

- Processing: Cereal grains are subjected to a variety of processing processes to remove the glucose-rich components:
  - Milling/Grinding: Milling or grinding operations are used on rice and wheat grains to remove the outer husk and retrieve the starchy endosperm, which contains glucose-rich carbohydrates.
  - Drying: Grain is dried to minimize moisture content, which assists in the strand avoiding spoiling.

2. Sugarcane: - Harvesting: Sugarcane is harvested when it reaches maturity, which is usually between 12 and 18 months after planting. The stalks are harvested by cutting them near the

ground. This may be done by hand or with mechanized harvesters that remove the stalks from the leaves.

- Sugarcane processing involves multiple stages to extract and refine the glucose-rich juice:
  - Crushing: Sugarcane stalks are crushed to obtain the juice, which contains sugar and other components.
  - Clarification: To eliminate contaminants and suspended materials, the extracted juice is treated with lime or other chemicals.
  - Evaporation and Boiling: To crystallize the sugars, the cleared juice is concentrated by evaporation and heat.
  - Centrifugation: The resultant sugar crystals are centrifuged to remove them from the syrup, giving raw sugar.
  - Refining: Raw sugar may be processed further to eliminate impurities and create refined white sugar.

3. Sugar Beets: - Harvesting: Sugar beets are root crops that are harvested when they reach maturity, which is normally after 90 to 120 days of development. Mechanical harvesters with blades or lifting mechanisms are often used to extract beets from the ground.

- Processing: Sugar beetroot processing entails multiple stages to extract and refine the glucose-rich juice:
  - Slicing: Sugar beets are gathered and cut into tiny pieces.
  - Extraction: The sliced beets go through a diffusion process in which hot water extracts the sugar from the chips.
  - Clarification and Evaporation: The extracted juice is clarified to eliminate contaminants and then evaporated to concentrate it.
  - Crystallisation: After boiling the concentrated juice, sugar crystals form and are removed from the syrup.
  - Refining: The raw sugar crystals may be processed to yield refined white sugar.

These are only a few examples of glucose-rich crop harvesting and processing procedures. Specific strategies may differ depending on crop variety, geographical area, and technology improvements. The purpose of these procedures is to effectively extract the glucose-rich components and purify them into useable forms, providing an essential source of energy for a wide range of culinary and industrial uses.

Understanding the impact of food processing on glucose

Depending on the exact processing procedures used, food processing may have various effects on the glucose level of meals. Here are some crucial points to consider about the effect of food processing on glucose:

1. Concentration and Availability: Food processing may concentrate or release glucose from its natural sources, making it easier for the body to digest and absorb. Juicing, pureeing, and grinding, for example, may break down the cellular structures of fruits and vegetables, releasing the glucose locked inside the plant cells. This may improve glucose availability and make it simpler for the body to digest and absorb.

2. Cooking procedures: The glucose content of meals may be affected by different cooking procedures. Boiling or steaming starchy meals such as potatoes, rice, or pasta, for example, may gelatinize their starches, making the glucose more available for digestion. Longer cooking durations or higher temperatures, on the other hand, might result in the breakdown of complex carbs into simpler sugars, thereby increasing the glucose concentration.

3. Added Sugars: Sugars, sweeteners, or syrups are often used in food processing to improve flavor, texture, or shelf life. These added sugars have the potential to considerably raise the glucose content of processed meals. It is crucial to remember that eating meals rich in added sugars may lead to health problems including obesity and metabolic diseases.

4. Fibre Content: Food processing may impact fiber content, which can affect glucose absorption and digestion. Dietary fiber, particularly soluble fiber, may assist to manage blood sugar levels by slowing glucose absorption. Processes that remove or decrease fiber content, such as refining grains or removing fruit skins, may result in quicker glucose absorption.

5. Glycemic Index: meal preparation may affect a meal's glycemic index (GI), which assesses how rapidly a food increases blood glucose levels. Processing procedures that break down complex carbs into simpler sugars may raise the GI of meals, causing blood sugar levels to rise more quickly. those with a high GI have a faster glucose reaction, while those with a low GI have a slower glucose release.

6. nutritional Loss: Some processing procedures, such as prolonged heating, might result in nutritional loss, including vitamins and minerals involved in glucose metabolism. It is critical to assess the overall nutritional content of processed meals since nutrient deficits might impair the body's capacity to use and regulate glucose adequately.

It is important to remember that the effect of food processing on glucose varies greatly depending on the particular food, processing procedures, and individual dietary context. It is best to prioritize whole, minimally processed foods and to examine the nutritional value, added sugars, and fiber content when purchasing processed food items to make educated decisions.

Chapter 4: Fueling Our Cells

The metabolic pathways of glucose utilization in the human body

Glucose, being a key source of energy, travels through many metabolic pathways in the human body before being used effectively. Let's look at the major metabolic processes involved in glucose utilization:

1. Glycolysis: Glycolysis is the first stage in the metabolism of glucose that happens in the cytoplasm of cells. Glucose is broken down into two molecules of pyruvate in this process. This process comprises a series of enzyme events that result in the production of a modest quantity of ATP (adenosine triphosphate) and NADH (nicotinamide adenine dinucleotide).

2. Pyruvate Dehydrogenase Complex (PDC): When there is enough oxygen, pyruvate from glycolysis reaches the mitochondria. The pyruvate dehydrogenase complex converts pyruvate to acetyl-CoA before proceeding to the next step. This phase connects glycolysis to the citric acid cycle (sometimes referred to as the Krebs cycle).

3. Citric Acid Cycle (Krebs Cycle): Within the mitochondria, acetyl-CoA enters the citric acid cycle. Acetyl-CoA is further broken down in this cycle, releasing CO_2 and producing ATP, NADH, and FADH2 (flavin adenine dinucleotide).

4. Oxidative Phosphorylation and the Electron Transport Chain (ETC): NADH and FADH2, which are created during glycolysis and the citric acid cycle, transport electrons to the inner mitochondrial membrane's electron transport chain. This mechanism creates a proton gradient through a sequence of electron transfer events, which drives ATP production via oxidative phosphorylation. ATP is the body's principal energy currency.

5. Gluconeogenesis: The process by which glucose is synthesized from non-carbohydrate precursors such as amino acids and glycerol is known as gluconeogenesis. It mostly affects the liver and, to a lesser degree, the kidneys. Gluconeogenesis aids in the maintenance of steady blood glucose levels during fasting or times of minimal carbohydrate consumption.

Glycogen Synthesis and Glycogenolysis: Excess glucose in the body may be turned to glycogen by glycogenesis, which occurs largely in the liver and muscles. Glycogen is a kind of glucose storage that may be broken down back into glucose through glycogenolysis when the body wants an immediate energy source.

7. Lipogenesis: When the body's immediate energy demands are met, surplus glucose may be turned into fatty acids through lipogenesis. These fatty acids may be stored in adipose tissue as triglycerides for long-term energy storage.

The hexose monophosphate shunt, often known as the pentose phosphate route, is an alternate method for glucose metabolism. It produces NADPH, a reducing agent needed for a variety of cellular functions including fatty acid synthesis and antioxidant defense.

These metabolic pathways work together to allow the body to use glucose effectively for energy generation, blood glucose management, and energy storage for future requirements. The balance between these pathways is closely maintained to maintain energy homeostasis and the appropriate functioning of the body's numerous tissues and organs.

Glucose and its Relationship with Lin in managing blood sugar levels

Glucose and insulin are critical in the regulation of blood sugar levels in the human body. Here's a rundown of their interaction and how they collaborate to maintain glucose homeostasis:

1. Glucose Regulation: Glucose is a sugar that cells use as their major source of energy. Carbohydrates are broken down into glucose during digestion and released into the circulation when we ingest them. Because high blood glucose levels may be harmful to one's health, the body has systems in place to control glucose levels within a small range.

2. Insulin Secretion: Insulin is a hormone generated by the pancreas's beta cells. Its primary function is to control glucose metabolism. When blood glucose levels rise after a meal, the pancreas responds by releasing insulin into the circulation.

3. Insulin and Glucose absorption: Insulin facilitates glucose absorption by acting on many tissues, including muscle, liver, and fat cells. It interacts with particular insulin receptors on the cell surface, causing a series of intracellular actions to occur. This mechanism causes glucose transporters, notably GLUT4, to move from intracellular compartments to the cell membrane. As a consequence, glucose enters cells more effectively.

4. Glucose Storage: Once within the cells, glucose may be used to produce energy or saved for later use. Glucose is turned into glycogen in muscle and liver cells by glycogenesis, a process

aided by insulin. Glycogen is a readily available type of glucose storage. Insulin also prevents glycogenolysis, which is the breakdown of glycogen into glucose.

5. Gluconeogenesis Inhibition: Insulin inhibits gluconeogenesis or the creation of glucose from non-carbohydrate sources such as amino acids and glycerol. Insulin helps to maintain lower blood glucose levels by lowering the liver's glucose production.

Insulin stimulates lipid synthesis and storage in adipose tissue by increasing fatty acid absorption and decreasing lipolysis, the breakdown of stored lipids. When blood glucose levels are high, this mechanism helps channel excess glucose away from adipose tissue, limiting excessive fat mobilization.

7. Feedback Loop: As blood glucose levels fall, insulin production decreases to avoid hypoglycemia (low blood sugar). This feedback loop maintains glucose metabolism in balance and avoids excessive insulin release.

Diabetes patients may have impaired insulin production (Type 1 diabetes) or insulin resistance (Type 2 diabetes). The usual glucose-insulin connection is disrupted, resulting in increased blood glucose levels. Diabetes management often includes drugs, lifestyle changes, and, in certain circumstances, insulin treatment to properly maintain blood sugar levels.

Understanding the link between glucose and insulin is essential for maintaining blood sugar control and avoiding the risks of persistent hyperglycemia. Regular blood glucose testing, suitable food choices, physical exercise, and adherence to prescription insulin regimens (where required) are all critical for diabetes management and general health.

The vital role of glucose in brain function and cognitive processes

Glucose is the major fuel source for the brain's energy demands and plays an important role in brain function. Here are a few essential points emphasizing the importance of glucose in brain function and cognitive processes:

1. Energy Source: Because the brain is a highly metabolically active organ, it needs a steady source of energy to operate properly. Brain cells prefer glucose as an energy source. ATP (adenosine triphosphate), the chemical that supplies energy for cellular functions, is produced when glucose is metabolized through glycolysis and subsequent pathways. To meet its energy requirements, the brain requires a constant supply of glucose.

2. Glucose transfer: Specific glucose transporters, such as GLUT1, promote glucose transfer across the blood-brain barrier. These transporters guarantee that glucose is constantly delivered from the circulation to the brain. The brain's capacity to properly use glucose is critical for sustaining optimal cognitive function.

3. Memory and Learning: The availability of glucose is related to memory formation and learning processes. According to research, maintaining steady blood glucose levels improves memory capacity and cognitive functioning. Cognitive activities such as attention, memory recall, and decision-making might be hampered when glucose levels are low.

4. Neuronal Activity: Glucose is utilized not just for energy generation, but also for neurotransmitter synthesis and neuronal activity maintenance. Neurotransmitters such as glutamate, dopamine, and serotonin are required for brain cell communication. Glucose metabolism produces the precursors required for neurotransmitter production, which influences neuronal signaling and general brain function.

5. Glucose Metabolism and Brain Health: Impaired glucose metabolisms, such as diabetes or insulin resistance, may be harmful to brain health. Chronically high blood sugar levels or insulin resistance may cause inflammation, oxidative stress, and brain cell damage, thus raising the risk of cognitive decline and neurodegenerative illnesses.

6. Brain Development: Glucose availability throughout important brain development phases is necessary for optimal neuronal growth, synaptogenesis, and neural network formation. Adequate glucose supply is required for adequate brain growth and good cognitive performance later in life, especially during fetal development and early childhood.

7. Neurological Disorders: Glucose imbalance has been linked to several neurological conditions. Alzheimer's disease, for example, is a neurodegenerative condition characterized by poor glucose metabolism in the brain. According to research, impaired glucose utilization may contribute to the advancement of neurodegenerative disorders.

In general, glucose is essential for brain function, cognitive processing, memory, and general brain health. Maintaining stable blood glucose levels via a well-balanced diet, frequent physical exercise, and good lifestyle habits are critical for optimal brain function and lowering the risk of cognitive deficits and neurological illnesses.

Chapter 5: Sweet Science

Investigating the chemistry of glucose in food preparation and cooking

The chemistry of glucose influences several elements of food preparation and cooking, including flavor, texture, browning responses, and nutritional changes. Here are some major features of glucose chemistry in food preparation:

1. Sweetness: Glucose is a naturally occurring sugar that adds to many meals' sweet flavors. The inclusion of glucose in food preparation may improve the impression of sweetness and balance the overall flavor profile. The sweet taste of glucose is determined by its molecular structure and interaction with taste receptors on the tongue.

2. Maillard Browning: Glucose contributes to Maillard browning processes, which occur when sugars react at high temperatures with amino acids or proteins. This process imparts a pleasant golden-brown color to cooked meals, increases flavor, and adds depth. Glucose may operate as a reducing sugar, supplying the carbonyl groups required for Maillard reactions, which result in the creation of flavor chemicals and odors.

3. Caramelization: When glucose is cooked to higher temperatures, it caramelizes. The breakdown of glucose molecules results in the creation of new compounds with distinctive caramel flavors and rich brown color. Caramelization produces the rich flavors found in caramel sauces, sweets, and certain baked items.

4. Texture and Moisture: Glucose can affect the texture and moisture content of meals. In baking, glucose serves as a humectant, attracting and holding moisture to help keep baked goods soft and fresh. It may also help to tenderize and moisten some confectionery goods like marshmallows and fudge.

5. Crystallisation: The propensity of glucose to form crystals influences the texture of some food items. Glucose syrup is often used in confectionery to regulate the development of sugar crystals, reducing undesired graininess in sweets or frostings. The presence of glucose creates a smoother texture by inhibiting sugar crystallization.

6. Fermentation: During the fermentation processes of baking and brewing, glucose acts as a substrate for yeast and other microbes. Yeast metabolizcreatese creates carbon creates, which enables the dough to rise and gives bread and other baked items a light, airy quality. Glucose fermentation also aids in the formation of flavors and fragrances in fermented foods and drinks.

7. Nutritional Changes: The cooking procedure has the potential to alter the availability and digestion of glucose in meals. Heat and cooking processes may break down complex carbs into simpler sugars such as glucose, making them more digestible and absorbable. This may lead to an enhanced glycemic response, which causes blood sugar levels to rise quicker. Furthermore, overcooking or extended heating may cause glucose and other carbohydrates to break down, resulting in changes in flavor, texture, and nutritional value.

Chefs and cooks may alter flavors, textures, and appearance in their culinary creations by understanding the chemistry of glucose in food preparation and cooking. It also sheds light on the nutritional changes that occur during cooking and may aid in the optimization of cooking processes to maximize the intended sensory qualities of meals.

The Maillard reaction and its connection to the browning of glucose-containing foods

When subjected to heat, the Maillard reaction is a complicated sequence of chemical events that occur between reducing carbohydrates such as glucose and amino acids or proteins. It is in charge of browning, fragrance, and flavor development in a variety of foods during cooking and processing. Here's a quick rundown of the Maillard reaction and how it relates to the browning of glucose-containing foods:

1. The Maillard process starts with the condensation of reducing sugar, such as glucose, with an amino group (-NH2) from an amino acid or protein. This condensation results in the formation of a glycosylamine intermediate. The intermediate is subsequently subjected to a succession of rearrangement, fragmentation, and polymerization events, which results in the synthesis of a diverse spectrum of flavor compounds, pigments, and volatile molecules.

2. Browning: Browning of food is one of the most apparent results of the Maillard process. When glucose participates in the Maillard process, it functions as a reducing sugar by supplying the reaction with a carbonyl group. As the Maillard reaction develops, melanoidin's are formed, which are responsible for the distinctive brown color of cooked meals.

3. Flavour and scent Development: The Maillard reaction produces a large number of volatile chemicals that add to food scent and flavor richness. Furans, pyrazines, thiophenes, and other chemicals provide appealing roasted, nutty, toasted, and savory flavors. The flavor is

determined by the amino acid and sugar types used in the reaction, as well as the reaction circumstances.

4. Temperature and Time: The Maillard process is temperature-dependent, with higher temperatures increasing the rate. At various temperature ranges, different reactions occur, resulting in the creation of particular flavor compounds. The Maillard reaction develops gradually over time, and longer cooking may result in deeper browning and more intense flavors.

5. Moisture and pH: The pH of the food system might affect the Maillard process. In general, alkaline circumstances accelerate the process, while acidic conditions may impede or change the reaction. Furthermore, moisture concentration influences the Maillard process. Excessive moisture may limit the Maillard process, whereas insufficient moisture might stimulate it.

6. Culinary Applications: Many culinary dishes benefit from the Maillard process. It gives seared meats, roasted coffee beans, toasted bread, grilled vegetables, and baked items their attractive color flavor. To achieve the appropriate browning and land flavorlopment, chefs and cooks often regulate the Maillard reaction by adjusting cooking temperatures, durations, and ingredient combinations.

While the Maillard reaction adds to the pleasant flavors and fragrances seen in cooked meals, excessive browning may result in the development of potentially hazardous chemicals such as acrylamide in high-starch foods cooked at high temperatures. To balance the favorable benefits of the Maillard reaction while minimizing the creation of unwanted byproducts, moderation,n, and proper cooking procedures are required.

Overall, the Maillard reaction is a complicated chemical process that happens during cooking between glucose and amino acids or proteins, resulting in the creation of browning, flavor, and fragrance in glucose-containing foods. Understanding the parameters that govern the Maillard reaction enables chefs and cooks to make a variety of delectable and aesthetically attractive foods.

Chapter 6: The Dark Side of Sweetness

The health implications of excessive glucose consumption

Excess glucose intake, especially in the form of added sugars and highly refined carbs, may have several detrimental health consequences. Here are some of the major health risks related to high glucose consumption:

1. Weight Gain and Obesity: Excessive glucose consumption may lead to weight gain and obesity. High-added sugar consumption, which s often found in sugary drinks, processed meals, and sweets, gives extra calories with little nutritious benefit. These extra calories might cause an imbalance in energy intake and expenditure, which can contribute to weight gain over time.

2. Increased chance of Type 2 Diabetes: Consuming excessive quantities of glucose regularly might raise the chance of acquiring type 2 diabetes. Excessive glucose consumption overwhelms the body's insulin response, resulting in insulin resistance. Insulin resistance may damage the body's capacity to control blood sugar levels over time, resulting in high blood glucose levels and the development of type 2 diabetes.

3. Poor oral Health: Excessive glucose intake, particularly in the form of sweet meals and drinks, may lead to poor oral health. Bacteria in the mouth consume sugar, generating acids that erode tooth enamel and cause tooth decay and cavities.

Excessive glucose intake has been related to an increased risk of chronic illnesses such as heart disease, some malignancies, and metabolic syndrome. Diets heavy in added sugars and refined carbohydrates have been linked to higher triglyceride levels, lower HDL cholesterol levels, higher blood pressure, and chronic inflammation, all of which are risk factors for these diseases.

5. Blood Sugar Fluctuations: Eating a lot of glucose-rich meals, particularly those with a high glycemic index, may produce fast rises in blood sugar levels followed by dips. These swings might cause weariness, irritation, and appetite. They may also lead to insulin resistance and reduced glucose tolerance in the long run.

6. Nutritional Imbalances: Glucose-rich foods, such as sugary snacks and drinks, often lack vital elements such as vitamins, minerals, and fiber. If these glucose-rich meals replace more nutrient-dense alternatives in the diet, they may lead to nutritional imbalances and deficits.

7. Effect on Metabolic Health: Excessive glucose intake may harm metabolic health indicators. High glucose consumption may lead to higher triglyceride levels, reduced HDL cholesterol levels, increased LDL cholesterol levels, and increased inflammatory indicators, all of which are risk factors for cardiovascular disease.

It's worth noting that naturally occurring glucose in healthy foods like fruits, vegetables, and whole grains is usually accompanied by fiber, vitamins, minerals, and phytochemicals, making these sources better alternatives than added sugars and highly processed diets. Moderation, balanced eating habits, and the intake of nutrient-dense foods are essential for maintaining a healthy diet and reducing the health hazards associated with excessive glucose consumption.

Understanding the link between glucose and obesity, diabetes, and other metabolic disorders

The link between glucose and obesity, diabetes, and other metabolic illnesses is complicated and diverse. The following is an explanation of the relationship between glucose and these conditions:

1. Obesity: Excess glucose intake, especially added sugars and highly processed carbs, may lead to weight gain and obesity. Glucose is an energy source that, if ingested in excess, may be stored as glycogen in the liver and muscles. When glycogen reserves are depleted, extra glucose is turned into fat through a process known as lipogenesis. Weight gain and obesity result from the increase of fat deposits over time. Furthermore, excessive glucose intake may lead to increased hunger, cravings, and a predilection for calorie-dense meals, encouraging weight gain.

2. Type 2 Diabetes: Type 2 diabetes is distinguished by insulin resistance, a disease in which cells become less receptive to insulin activity, resulting in high blood sugar levels. Excess glucose intake, particularly in the form of added sugars and refined carbs, may lead to insulin resistance development. High glucose consumption causes blood sugar increases, requiring the pancreas to generate more insulin to manage glucose levels. The continual need for insulin may lead to decreased insulin sensitivity and the development of insulin resistance over time. As a consequence, glucose is not properly absorbed by cells, resulting in the high blood sugar levels associated with type 2 diabetes.

3. Metabolic Syndrome: A metabolic syndrome is a group of disorders that includes obesity, high blood pressure, high blood sugar levels, and abnormal lipid profiles (high triglycerides and low HDL cholesterol). Through a variety of ways, excessive glucose intake may lead to the development of metabolic syndrome. High glucose levels may cause insulin resistance, which can promote belly fat storage, raise blood pressure, and disturb lipid metabolism. Furthermore, glucose-rich meals, particularly those with a high glycemic index, may induce fast increases in blood sugar levels, leading to metabolic disruptions and an increased risk of metabolic syndrome.

4. Cardiovascular Disease: Excess glucose intake might be harmful to one's cardiovascular health. Diets rich in added sugars and refined carbohydrates have been linked to higher triglyceride levels, lower HDL cholesterol levels, higher LDL cholesterol levels, and higher inflammatory indicators. These variables lead to atherosclerosis (hardening and constriction of the arteries) and an increased risk of cardiovascular disorders such as heart disease and stroke.

5. Non-alcoholic Fatty Liver Disease (NAFLD): NAFLD is a disease in which fat accumulates in the liver but is not caused by excessive alcohol intake. Excess glucose intake, especially added sweets, may contribute to the development of NAFLD. When the liver's ability to store glucose as glycogen is exceeded, the surplus glucose is turned into fatty acids, which accumulate in the liver. This, in turn, may cause inflammation, liver damage, and the advancement of NAFLD.

While excessive glucose intake may contribute to these disorders, the total dietary pattern, including food consumption, physical activity levels, and hereditary variables, all play key roles in their development. A healthy body weight, a balanced diet, moderate sugar intake, regular physical exercise, and maintaining a healthy body weight are all important for lowering the risk of obesity, diabetes, and other metabolic diseases.

Strategies for maintaining a balanced glucose intake and promoting overall health

Maintaining a healthy glucose intake is critical for general health and avoiding the harmful implications of high glucose consumption. Here are some tips to help you reach a healthy glucose consumption and improve your overall health:

1. Prioritise entire Foods: Include entire foods in your diet such as fruits, vegetables, whole grains, lean meats, and healthy fats. These meals provide important nutrients, fiber, and a balanced combination of carbs, including glucose, as well as other beneficial substances. Whole foods have a lower glycemic index, which means they affect blood sugar levels more slowly and steadily.

2. Limit Added Sugars: Limit your intake of meals and drinks rich in added sugars. Sugary beverages, pastries, candies, and processed meals all include added sugars, which give empty calories with no nutritious benefit. Look for hidden sources of added sugars on food labels, such as corn syrup, fructose, sucrose, or any ingredient ending in "-ose." Choose naturally sweetened foods or, as an alternative, use tiny quantities of natural sweeteners such as honey or maple syrup.

3. Include Complex carbs in Your Diet: Include complex carbs in your diet, such as whole grains (e.g., brown rice, quinoa, whole wheat), legumes, and starchy vegetables. These meals include higher fiber, which slows glucose digestion and absorption, assisting in the maintenance of stable blood sugar levels. They also give extra nutrients and aid with satiety.

4. Combine carbs with Protein and Fat: When eating carbs, pair them with protein and healthy fats. This combination may assist to decrease the absorption of glucose into the circulation, reducing blood sugar rises. Have an apple with a handful of almonds, or whole-grain bread with avocado and eggs.

5. Practise meal Control: Watch your meal sizes to prevent consuming too much glucose. When ingested in high numbers, even nutritious meals might lead to an unbalanced glucose intake. To guide your dietary choices, use measurement equipment or get acquainted with portion amounts.

6. Stress the Importance of Regular Physical Exercise: Regular physical exercise may help manage blood sugar levels and enhance insulin sensitivity. Exercise increases glucose absorption by the muscles, lowering insulin demand. To maximize the advantages, combine aerobic activity with strength training.

7. Drink lots of water throughout the day to stay hydrated. Proper hydration benefits general health and may help avoid overeating or snacking, both of which can lead to an unbalanced glucose intake.

8. Monitor Blood Sugar Levels: If you have diabetes or are concerned about your blood sugar levels, work with your doctor to successfully monitor and control your glucose levels. Regular monitoring, medication management (if necessary), and lifestyle changes may all assist to keep glucose levels in check.

9. Seek practitioner Help: If you have special health issues or dietary requirements, talk to a qualified nutritionist or healthcare practitioner. They can provide you with personalized advice and suggestions based on your specific scenario.

Remember that healthy glucose consumption is just one part of total wellness. To achieve maximum well-being, it is critical to take a holistic approach that includes a well-balanced diet, frequent physical exercise, stress management, enough sleep, and other good lifestyle practices.

Chapter 7: Beyond the Palate

Exploring the non-edible applications of glucose in industries such as pharmaceuticals, cosmetics, and biofuels

Because of its varied qualities, glucose is used in a variety of sectors outside of its position as a food carbohydrate. Here are some examples of non-edible glucose uses in sectors such as medicines, cosmetics, and biofuels:

1. Pharmaceuticals: Glucose is an essential component in the manufacture of several medicinal drugs. It is often employed as an excipient in tablet formulations, providing stability and functioning as a filler or binder. Glucose is also used as an energy source in intravenous (IV) solutions and parenteral nutrition for individuals who are unable to take meals orally. Glucose derivatives are also used in the production of antibiotics, anti-inflammatory medicines, and other medicinal substances.

2. Cosmetics: In the cosmetics business, glucose and its derivatives are highly prized components. Because of their moisturizing and humectant characteristics, they may be found in a variety of skincare, haircare, and personal care products. Glucose is a moisturizing substance that attracts and holds moisture in the skin and hair. It also aids in the smooth texture and emollient properties of cosmetic compositions.

3. Biofuels: Glucose is used in the manufacturing of biofuels, notably bioethanol. Microorganisms such as yeast digest glucose or other sugar-rich feedstocks to produce bioethanol. Glucose generated from agricultural products such as maize or sugarcane may be transformed enzymatically into ethanol, which is utilized as a sustainable fuel additive or as a direct substitute for petrol in specific applications.

4. Bioplastics and Biomaterials: Glucose may be used to make bioplastics and biomaterials, which are more ecologically friendly than typical petroleum-based plastics and materials. Polylactic acid (PLA), a glucose-based polymer, may be generated from renewable sources and has uses in packaging, biomedical devices, and other sectors. When compared to traditional plastics, these materials are biodegradable and have lesser environmental implications.

5. Biotechnology and Biomedical Research: Glucose is an important food source of energy in a variety of biotechnological and biomedical applications. Glucose is extensively utilized as a

carbon source in cell culture and fermentation procedures to promote the development and metabolic activity of microorganisms and human cells. It supplies the energy required for cell growth as well as the creation of recombinant proteins, antibiotics, and other bioactive substances.

6. Diagnostic Testing: Glucose is commonly used in diagnostic testing, notably for measuring blood sugar levels with glucose meters or laboratory procedures. These tests are critical for monitoring and controlling diabetes, which is defined by poor glucose regulation. Glucose is also used in various diagnostic procedures to determine metabolic health and insulin sensitivity, such as glucose tolerance tests.

7. Wound Healing and Tissue Engineering: The use of glucose-based materials and hydrogels in wound healing and tissue engineering. These materials may act as a scaffold for cell development and help regenerate damaged tissues. Glucose is often included in biomaterials to enhance cell viability and metabolic activity during the repair and regeneration of tissues.

Glucose's adaptability goes beyond its position as a dietary carbohydrate. Its use in medicines, cosmetics, biofuels, and other sectors demonstrates its importance in a variety of scientific and commercial endeavors. In these and other sectors, ongoing research and innovation are looking for novel and sustainable applications for glucose.

Glucose as a source of renewable energy and its potential environmental benefits

Glucose has a lot of promise as a renewable energy source with a lot of environmental advantages. Here's a look at its position as a renewable energy source and the environmental benefits that come with it:

1. Biofuel Production: Through processes such as fermentation, glucose may be turned into biofuels such as bioethanol. In certain instances, bioethanol made from glucose may be used as a sustainable fuel additive or as an alternative to petrol. Bioethanol generated from glucose has various environmental benefits over fossil fuels. It is made from renewable biomass, decreasing reliance on limited fossil fuel stocks. Bioethanol emits less greenhouse gas emissions, such as carbon dioxide, into the environment when burnt than regular petrol, helping to mitigate climate change.

2. Lower Carbon Footprint: The development of glucose-based biofuels may assist lower the transportation sector's total carbon footprint. Because glucose is obtained from biomass sources such as crops or organic waste, the carbon dioxide released during its burning is fundamentally part of the natural carbon cycle. The carbon dioxide produced by biofuel burning

is reabsorbed by plants during photosynthesis, resulting in a closed carbon cycle. In contrast to fossil fuels, which release carbon dioxide from long-buried carbon deposits, glucose-based biofuels are more sustainable and carbon-neutral.

3. Renewable Energy Storage: Glucose may also be used to store renewable energy. Glucose may be turned into electrical energy using techniques such as enzymatic or microbial fuel cells. This has the potential to offer a way to store and use renewable energy provided by sources such as solar or wind power. Glucose-based energy storage devices may assist balance intermittent renewable energy supplies by offering a regular and predictable power source.

4. Waste Valorization: Glucose may be produced from a variety of biomass sources, such as agricultural leftovers, food waste, and energy crops. Utilizing these biomass sources to manufacture glucose-based biofuels not only offers sustainable energy but also aids in waste material valorization. It decreases the environmental effect of waste disposal and contributes to a more sustainable waste management system by diverting biomass waste from landfills and transforming it into a useful energy supply.

5. Lower Air Pollution: When compared to fossil fuels, the burning of glucose-based biofuels generates less hazardous pollutants such as sulfur dioxide, nitrogen oxides, and particle matter. These contaminants lead to air pollution, smog formation, and negative health consequences. It is feasible to minimize air pollution and enhance air quality by replacing or combining fossil fuels with biofuels generated from glucose, benefitting both human health and the environment.

6. Sustainable Agriculture: Growing biomass for glucose production may help to encourage sustainable agricultural practices. Energy crops such as sugarcane, maize, and switchgrass may be farmed in an environmentally responsible way. These crops may help to conserve soil, sequester carbon, and preserve biodiversity. Furthermore, expanding the agricultural sector to incorporate energy crops may give farmers extra revenue prospects while also supporting rural economies.

While glucose-based biofuels provide environmental advantages, their total sustainability and effect are dependent on a variety of variables such as biomass supply, growing practices, land usage, and manufacturing procedures. To maximize the environmental advantages of glucose as a renewable energy source, ethical sourcing, efficient manufacturing techniques, and a thorough life cycle analysis are required.

Innovations and Prospects for glucose utilization

Glucose utilization is still an active field of study and innovation, with intriguing promise for a variety of applications. Here are several glucose utilization advances and prospects:

1. Advanced Biofuels: Scientists are investigating advanced biofuel production processes that use glucose and other carbohydrates as feedstocks. Cellulosic biofuels, for example, utilize non-food biomass sources such as agricultural leftovers, specialized energy crops, and algae. Such developments may provide better fuel economy, lower greenhouse gas emissions, and a larger choice of feedstock possibilities for renewable energy generation by effectively converting glucose into biofuels.

2. Bioplastics and Biodegradable Materials: Bioplastics currently employ glucose-based polymers such as polylactic acid (PLA). However, continuing research focuses on improving their mechanical strength, thermal stability, and biodegradability. The development of glucose-derived polymers with enhanced performance properties has the potential to broaden their uses in a variety of sectors, including packaging, consumer products, and biomedical materials.

3. Biomedical Applications: The use of glucose-based materials and technology in biomedical applications such as drug delivery systems, tissue engineering, and regenerative medicine is being investigated. Researchers are looking at glucose-responsive drug delivery systems, which release medicine in response to glucose levels, allowing for targeted and controlled drug release for illnesses such as diabetes. To aid tissue regeneration and wound healing, glucose-based hydrogels and scaffolds are being produced.

4. Energy Storage: Glucose-based energy storage devices, such as glucose fuel cells, hold great potential as efficient and long-lasting energy storage solutions. These systems can directly convert glucose into electrical energy, making them suitable for use in portable electronics, implanted medical devices, and renewable energy storage. Advances in glucose fuel cell technology, such as the development of more efficient catalysts and electrode materials, have the potential to increase performance and expand deployment.

5. Sustainable Chemical Production: Glucose is a renewable starting material for the manufacture of a variety of chemicals and bioproducts. Bio-based fermentation technologies are being investigated by researchers to convert glucose into useful molecules such as organic acids, solvents, and platform chemicals. These environmentally friendly manufacturing techniques provide alternatives to typical petrochemical-based processes, lowering dependency on fossil resources and minimizing environmental consequences.

6. Glucose Monitoring and Personalised Nutrition: As wearable and non-invasive glucose monitoring technology progress, people may watch their glucose levels in real-time. When combined with artificial intelligence and personalized nutrition techniques, this might allow

people to make more educated food decisions based on their glucose reactions. Bringing glucose monitoring and a personalized diet together has the potential to improve health, manage chronic illnesses, and increase general well-being.

7. Sustainable Agriculture and Crop Improvement: Efforts are being made to improve the efficiency of glucose generation from biomass sources and to optimize energy crop farming. This includes the development of high-yielding, disease-resistant energy crop varieties, as well as the improvement of crop management practices and the use of precision agricultural technology. Such developments have the potential to contribute to sustainable agriculture, food security, and bioenergy production.

We may anticipate further innovations and breakthroughs in using glucose in many industries as research continues to enhance our knowledge of glucose and its possible uses. Sustainable and efficient processes, as well as the incorporation of glucose-based technology into numerous sectors, offer enormous potential for a more sustainable and bio-based future.

Chapter 8: The Sweet Symphony of Flavors

The role of glucose in enhancing and balancing flavors in culinary creations

Glucose is essential for increasing and balancing flavors in culinary creations. Glucose contributes to flavor formation in food in the following ways:

1. Increased Sweetness: Glucose is a naturally occurring sugar with a sweet flavor. When added to food, it increases the impression of sweetness, increasing the overall flavor profile. Glucose may be used to sweeten a variety of foods, including baked products, confectionery, sauces, and drinks.

2. Flavour Balancing: Glucose aids in flavor balance by counteracting excessive bitterness or acidity in particular components or recipes. It functions as a flavor enhancer, helping to soften or level off strong or harsh flavors. Chefs and cooks may produce a better taste balance by adding glucose, resulting in a more harmonious flavor profile.

3. Browning and Caramelization: Glucose contributes to the Maillard process, which results in browning and the production of complex flavors during cooking. When glucose interacts with amino acids at high temperatures, pleasant flavors, and fragrances such as nutty, toasted, and caramel overtones are produced. This response is what gives roasted meats, caramel sauces, and baked items their enticing flavors.

4. Texture Enhancement: Glucose may increase the texture of some culinary items, resulting in a more sensual experience. Glucose aids in the reduction of ice crystal formation in goods such as ice cream, sorbets, and frozen desserts, resulting in a smoother and creamier texture. It may also be used to provide chewiness or softness to sweets, jams, and confections.

5. Flavour Preservation: By functioning as a humectant, glucose may help retain the flavors of certain substances. It draws and holds moisture as a humectant, keeping food from drying out and maintaining natural flavors. This is especially useful in baked products, pastries, and other foods where flavor preservation is important.

6. Fermentation and Flavour Development: During fermentation, yeast and other microbes quickly eat glucose. Glucose serves as a source of energy for microbes in the fermentation of

bread, beer, wine, and other fermented goods, culminating in the synthesis of alcohol and different flavor compounds. This adds to the distinct flavors and fragrances of fermented foods and drinks.

While glucose helps to flavor development its use should be balanced and matched to individual culinary production. A well-balanced and tasty flavor profile is achieved by the concentration and mix of components, cooking processes, and personal preferences. Chefs and chefs often experiment with various sugars, including glucose, to establish the correct balance and improve the flavors of their culinary creations.

Exploring the art of pastry and confectionery through the lens of glucose

Glucose is used extensively in pastry and confectionery, bringing both utilitarian and artistic features to these culinary treats. In the field of pastry and confectionery, glucose is used as follows:

1. Sweetness and Texture: Glucose is a typical sweetener used in the manufacturing of pastries and confections. Its sweet flavor adds to the overall flavor profile of sweet delights, while its distinct molecular structure contributes to the desired texture. Glucose contributes to the smooth and creamy mouthfeel of items such as caramel, fudge, and nougat. It also prevents sugar crcrystallizationresulting in a soft and smooth texture in sweets and frostings.

2. Sugar Syrups and Fondants: A viscous and sweet syrup formed from glucose, glucose syrup, is an important component in many pastry and confectionery recipes. It is used in the production of sugar syrups, which provide moisture, sweetness, and gloss to cakes, pastries, and desserts. Glucose syrup is also an important ingredient in fondant, a malleable frosting used to cover cakes and make ornamental components. Fondant with glucose syrup has a smooth and elastic consistency, making it simpler to work with during cake decorating.

3. Improved Stability and Shelf Life: Glucose improves the stability and shelf life of pastries and confections. Glucose works as a humectant in baked products such as cakes, cookies, and bread, maintaining moisture and avoiding staling. This helps the items retain their freshness and suppleness over time. Glucose is also used to extend the shelf life of some confections, such as marshmallows and gummies, by preventing them from becoming dry or hard.

4. Caramelization and Browning: The Maillard reaction, which happens when glucose combines with amino acids, is critical in the pastry and confectionery arts. Browning and the creation of complex flavors in baked products, pastries, and caramel-based confections are caused by this

process. Glucose is essential in achieving the correct caramelization, which gives pastries a golden crust and confections a rich caramel flavor.

5. Binding Agent: In several pastry and confectionery recipes, glucose works as a binding agent. It holds compounds together and creates structure, particularly in nougat, marshmallows, and caramel sweets. Glucose supplies the requisite stickiness and binding characteristics that aid in the retention of form and texture in these confections.

6. Chocolatiering: Glucose is used in a variety of ways in the chocolate industry. It's a common component in chocolate fillings and ganaches, where it adds smoothness and texture. Glucose may also be included in chocolate recipes to assist manage crystallization and provide a smooth, glossy finish. Furthermore, glucose is used in the manufacture of confectionery coatings and glazes, which add shine and improve the texture of chocolate-covered sweets.

Exploring the art of pastry and confectionery through the perspective of glucose enables chefs, pastry chefs, and confectioners to produce a variety of delectable delicacies. Glucose is a versatile component that adds to the mastery of various culinary skills by boosting sweetness and texture, giving stability, and assisting in caramelization.

Experimenting with glucose in the kitchen: recipes, tips, and tricks

Experimenting with glucose in the kitchen may open up a world of possibilities for developing one-of-a-kind and delectable meals. Here are some glucose-inspired recipes, techniques, and methods to get you started:

1. Glucose Syrup: Make your glucose syrup in a pot by blending 1 cup of water and 12 cups of glucose powder. Stir the liquid over medium heat until the glucose powder dissolves completely. In a variety of recipes, use this syrup as a sweetener and moisture-retaining agent.

2. Caramel Sauce: In a saucepan, combine 1 cup of sugar, 14 cups of water, 2 teaspoons of butter, and 2 tablespoons of glucose syrup to make a thick and silky caramel sauce. Stir the liquid over medium heat until the sugar is completely dissolved. Cook, stirring occasionally, until the liquid becomes amber in color. Remove from the fire and gradually whisk in 12 cups of heavy cream until smooth. For added flavor, sprinkle with a touch of salt. Use this caramel sauce over ice cream, in pastries, or as a fruit dip.

3. Chewy Caramel Candies: In a saucepan, combine 1 cup of sugar, 12 cups of heavy cream, 12 cups of glucose syrup, 3 tablespoons of butter, and a teaspoon of salt. Stir continually over medium heat until the mixture registers 245°F (118°C) on a candy thermometer. Allow the mixture to cool fully on a prepared baking tray before cutting into individual candies.

4. Smooth Ice Cream: To enhance the smoothness and avoid crystallization, add a tiny quantity of glucose syrup (1-2 teaspoons) to your handmade ice cream base. The glucose syrup functions as an anti-crystallizing agent, making the ice cream smoother and creamier.

5. Pastry Glaze: In a saucepan, combine equal parts glucose syrup and water to make a glossy and tasty glaze for pastries. Heat the mixture over low heat until it reaches the consistency of a thin syrup. For a beautiful and professional finish, brush the glaze over freshly cooked pastries such as fruit tarts or danishes.

6. Marshmallows: To get a smooth and fluffy texture, use glucose syrup in your homemade marshmallow recipes. It contributes to stability by keeping the marshmallows from getting overly stiff or sticky.

7. Candy production: Glucose is an important element in candy production since it controls sugar crystallization and adds chewiness. Experiment using glucose in gummy, caramel, nougat, and other candy recipes to create the desired texture and consistency.

Tricks and tips:

- Working with glucose syrup may be sticky and difficult to correctly measure. Before measuring the syrup, carefully cover your measuring spoon or cup with nonstick cooking spray or immerse it in hot water to make it easier to handle.

- Glucose is hygroscopic, which means it draws and holds moisture. Store glucose powder or syrup in an airtight container in a cold, dry area to avoid clumping.

- In most recipes, glucose syrup may be substituted for corn syrup, however, flavor and texture may change somewhat.

- Begin with little quantities of glucose in your dishes and gradually increase as your taste preferences dictate. Because it may be rather sweet, be careful not to overshadow the flavors of the other components.

- A modest quantity of glucose syrup may assist avoid crystallization and provide a smooth caramel when caramelizing sugar.

When playing with glucose in the kitchen, remember to have fun and be creative. This ingredient's adaptability opens you with unlimited opportunities for producing tasty and one-of-a-kind gourmet masterpieces

Chapter 9: The Cultural Connection

The Cultural Link: Investigating Glucose in Culinary Traditions

Food and culture are inextricably linked, and the use of glucose in culinary traditions from throughout the world demonstrates the variety and originality of human gastronomy. Let's look at the cultural significance of glucose in diverse culinary traditions:

1. Asian Cuisine: Glucose-rich foods such as rice, rice noodles, and rice flour are common components in many Asian dishes. Traditional foods containing glucose include Chinese mooncakes, Thai mango sticky rice, and Japanese mochi. These scrumptious delights show the cultural importance of glucose-rich foods as well as the skill of making tasty snacks.

2. Middle Eastern Delights: Glucose is offeredilizeded in Middle Eastern cuisine in the form of date syrup or honey. These glucose-rich natural sweeteners are crucial in sweets such as baklava, halva, and Turkish delight. Glucose lends sweetness and texture to these classic delicacies, giving them a particular cultural character.

3. European Confections: Glucose is an important component of European candy traditions. Glucose is utilized to provide the correct texture, stability, and flavor in anything from French pastries like éclairs and macarons to Italian panettone and British fudge. European civilizations have evolved distinct confectionery methods that use the characteristics of glucose to make delectable treats.

4. Latin American Sweets: A variety of glucose-rich sweets and desserts may be found in Latin American cuisine. In Mexico, for example, popular delicacies such as dulce de leche, churros, and tres leches cake include glucose. Traditional sweets such as cajeta and alfajores are also made using glucose syrup. These confections highlight Latin American communities' cultural history and culinary ability.

5. Indian Sweets: Mithai, or glucose-rich sweets, are abundant in Indian cuisine. Gulab jamun, jalebi, barfi, and rasgulla are among these delights. Glucose, which is frequently obtained from milk solids and grains, offers the requisite sweetness, texture, and binding qualities for these classic Indian sweets.

6. African Delicacies: Glucose-rich components are employed in a range of traditional meals across Africa's different regions. In North African cuisine, for example, glucose may be found in

Moroccan pastries such as honey-drenched pastillas and sweet almond-filled gazelle horns. Glucose-rich foods such as plantains and yams arutilizeded in recipes such as fried plantain chips and yam fritters in Sub-Saharan Africa.

7. Indigenous Culinary Traditions: Glucose-rich foods have long been a part of indigenous culinary traditions across the globe. Glucose-rich foods link these cultures to their cultural origins and represent their profound understanding of local resources, from Native American corn-based sweets like popcorn balls and cornbread to South Pacific taro-based desserts.

Exploring glucose in culinary cultures reveals cultural legacy, innovation, and culinary skills created and honed through h years. These traditions on honourorur the flavors and textures provided by glucose, but they also develop a feeling of community, identity, and pride in the many cultures who embrace and use this crucial component in their cupracticesactise

Conclusion.

Finally, the exploration of the world of glucose showed its diverse function in culinary creativity, cultural traditions, and human health. Glucose has shown to be a versatile element that enriches our culinary experiences, from its molecular structure and qualities to its influence on flavor, texture, and sweetness.

We looked at how glucose functions as a critical source of energy in the human body, its relationship with insulin and blood sugar management, and its importance in brain function and cognitive activities. Furthermore, we investigated its natural origins, which include fruits, vegetables, and honey, and followed its journey from agricultural fields to our plates through harvesting, processing, and food preparation processes.

Glucose's cultural significance has been a fascinating trip as we uncovered its existence in culinary cultures throughout the globe. Glucose has played an important part in developing the different flavors, textures, and customs of each culture's culinary history, from Asian delicacies to Middle Eastern treats, European confections to Latin American sweets, and beyond.

We have also investigated non-edible applications of glucose in sectors such as medicines, cosmetics, and biofuels, emphasizing its flexibility and potential for novel use outside of the kitchen. Furthermore, we investigated the environmental advantages of glucose as a renewable energy source, demonstrating its potential for a sustainable future.

While it is important to manage glucose consumption to prevent health consequences, we explored ways for maintaining a healthy glucose intake while also improving general well-being. We can assure a balanced and healthy diet by knowing its influence on obesity, diabetes, and metabolic illnesses.

Finally, we investigated the chemistry of glucose in food preparation and cooking, learning about its function in the Maillard process and the browning of glucose-containing meals. We investigated the art of pastry and confectionery through the prism of glucose, learning how it enriches flavors, improves texture, and leads to mastery of these culinary arts.

The study of glucose has shown its importance as a component that crosses borders, cultures, and industries. It provides inspiration, cultural identity, and sustenance, improving our culinary experiences and linking us to our history, present, and future. Embracing and understanding the function of glucose may open up a world of culinary possibilities and boost your awareness of the complicated interaction between food, culture, and human health, whether you're a chef, a home cook, or just a food fan.